God Is in Control!

Cancer from a Patient/ Social Worker Perspective

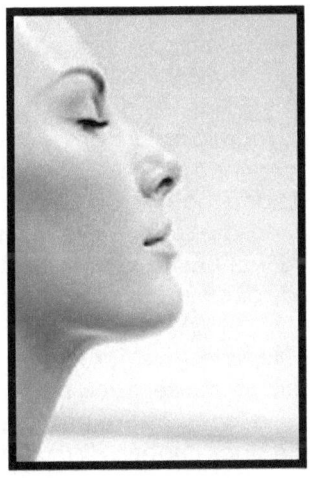

Kaye Elliott Leazier

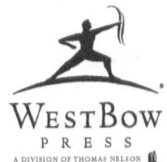

WestBow
PRESS
A DIVISION OF THOMAS NELSON

WestBow Press books may be ordered through
booksellers or by contacting:

WestBow Press
A Division of Thomas Nelson
1663 Liberty Drive
Bloomington, IN 47403
www.westbowpress.com
1-(866) 928-1240

ISBN: 978-1-4497-9208-4 (sc)
ISBN: 978-1-4497-9209-1 (e)
Library of Congress Control Number: 2013907103
Printed in the United States of America.

Scripture quotations taken from the New American
Standard Bible®, Copyright © 1960, 1962, 1963, 1968, 1971,
1972, 1973, 1975, 1977, 1995 by The Lockman Foundation.
Used by permission." (www.Lockman.org)

WestBow Press rev. date: 4/24/2013

Foreword by Dennis D. Frey, D.Th., President
Master's International School of Divinity

Dedication

This book is dedicated first and foremost to:
Jesus Christ, my Savior and Lord.

Then to:
Dean H. Elliott, my brother,
(January 3, 1945 – April 12, 2007)
who valiantly fought and lost his own battle
with brain cancer as I worked on this project.

and to:
Joseph L. Leazier, my husband,
who went through my battle with me,
while fighting his own battle with PTSD.

and finally to:
Dr. Dennis D. Frey, my brother in Christ,
without whose encouragement I
would never have completed this.

THANK YOU!

Foreword

Those who serve in the helping professions, whether in counseling, social work or Christian ministry, are universally persons who sincerely care about the needs of others. In their own unique way, these individuals give from an inner resource of sympathy and love. They invest in themselves years of education and training in order to meet the requirements of their chosen field. Beyond that, they polish their skills of insight and discernment in the everyday struggles of real life.

Most of us in the helping professions, while not immune to the difficulties and trauma of those we serve, for the most part study their ordeals from the outside. This makes us professional sympathizers not fellow participants. This is decidedly not the case with Kaye Leazier. She is a fellow participant.

After decades of serving others from the outside, without warning, she found herself in the crucible of a life and death struggle with a woman's most feared and hated biological enemy...breast cancer. Her personal journey into the "tunnel" as she calls it provides a rare opportunity to witness the way a care *giver* reacts when faced with being the care *receiver*. Her gift to thousands of women who have shared her journey and to the company of wonderful sympathizing women and men who serve in the helping professions is the story of her triumph as told in this book.

Kaye has been to the edge of the abyss, and has survived. However, she has not survived alone. She is a sterling example of what the Apostle Paul was speaking of when he said, "I know how to get along with humble means, and I also know how to live in prosperity; in any and every circumstance I have learned the secret of being filled and going hungry, both of having abundance and suffering need. I can do all things through Him who

strengthens me" (Philippians 4:12-13 NASV).
This is why she says, "God is in Control!"

Dennis D. Frey, Th.D,
President Master's International School of
Divinity
Evansville, Indiana

Preface

This is the author's personal journey from the finding of a suspicious spot in a routine mammogram to a year past her bilateral mastectomy. She shares some candid moments as well as insights from both a patient and social worker perspective. The book is educational as well as entertaining and is easy to read. You will feel both her pain and humor as you travel the road with her. So be ready to laugh and to cry. She is convinced God's hand was obvious throughout her ordeal and reminds believers to trust him and also to realize God remains in control. She includes two "what to do" and "what not to do" lists, one for a patient and one for a social worker.

This book was written to fulfill the writing project requirement of the Doctor of Biblical Studies degree for Master's International School of Divinity.

ALL SCRIPTURE is Quoted from the New American Standard Bible Unless otherwise stated.

All names except the author and her husband's have been camouflaged to protect the privacy of each individual. All persons represented are real people and known personally by the author.

The events and happenings represented in this paper are factual and personally experienced by the author.

Endnotes and Appendices are Included at the end of this paper to provide additional information.

Table of Contents

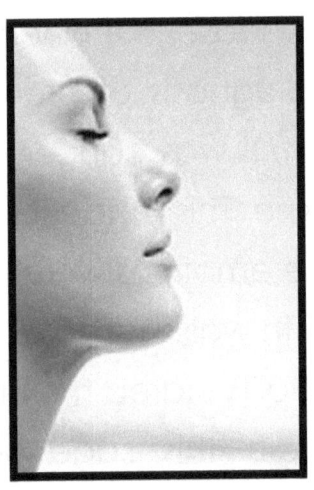

It's Just a Bump in the Road

So many emotions! This wasn't supposed to be the outcome. How can this be? What do I do now? What questions do I need to ask? I'm feeling numb. Brain, START WORKING!... Anyone who has heard a doctor say, "I'm sorry, it's cancer" understands this confusion. As a counselor and medical social worker, I have worked with numerous cancer patients and survivors. As a daughter I have lost two parents to this disease. But when I personally received the diagnosis of breast cancer it was all different. It was cancer... and it was happening to me. This made it a whole new experience. The emotions were raw, the fear was real, my faith was shaken and the reality of my own mortality stared me in the face.

Let me begin this saga with a little background. My family has a long history of cancer, so it is something I have dealt with before. I have lost aunts and uncles, on both sides to this disease, as well as cousins. My father died of lung cancer, after a short battle, when I was 40. The same year, my mother was diagnosed with breast cancer. Mom opted for a lumpectomy[1] and radiation[2]. The doctor told us, mom would probably die of something else before the cancer would ever come back. Wrong! Mom was cancer free for three years and then it came back with a vengeance. She fought bravely for a year before succumbing to the inevitable. Mom died in 2000, I received my diagnosis in 2005.

I have been a social worker for years, and worked in the medical field most of that time. I was used to dealing with illnesses. I have even had numerous health issues myself over the years, but this diagnosis was just a little too raw and too soon after my mom's death. But I am getting ahead of myself here, so let me back up a little bit.

In September of 2004, my husband was forced into an early and unwanted retirement. We were not ready for this either emotionally or financially; so the stress began. Don't let anyone tell you stress does not affect your health! [3] Realizing we were under an enormous amount of stress and anxiety, I decided we had to become healthier. So I prayed about it and asked God to get me healthy so I could be of better service for Him. The summer of 2005, I started cooking healthier and my husband and I were consciously changing our lifestyles. We were losing weight, gaining some energy and starting to get over the shock of his unemployment status. We were beginning to think we would make it after all. God was definitely in control.

Now, God does work in mysterious ways. Remember I prayed and asked him to get me healthy. Well, God knew there was a cancer growing inside me that was going to mess up my plans. I went for a routine mammogram[4], and was surprised when my doctor called and asked if the hospital had called me yet. When I said no, she explained the radiologist[5] had seen a suspicious area and wanted a follow-up ultrasound[6]. The machine and computer did not spot anything unusual, but the radiologist spotted something he didn't like. Okay, no big deal, I have fibrous cysts and so I often have suspicious areas. So I waited for the hospital to call. When they did, they told me the regular ultrasound technician was on vacation. I could wait until she returned, or could come in with the temporary technician, but he was male. Since, I believe medical personnel are professionals, I chose to schedule as soon as possible. I just wanted to get it done and over with. I had better things to do, so I thought. James 4:15 tells us otherwise; "Instead,, *you ought* to say, "If the Lord wills, we shall live and also do this or that." I forgot I was not the one in control.

The day of the ultrasound, I wasn't the least bit worried. I expected it to show nothing was out of the ordinary. The male technician came and got me from the waiting room and explained he worked in radiology, at the Marquette Hospital, which was a bigger hospital than the one I was getting the ultrasound at. He explained what the radiologist had seen and what he would be looking for. He also explained he wanted to do a special procedure to get a better picture, so had asked the mammography technician to assist. Once the procedure started I asked questions, so he moved the screen so I could see it. The special procedure consisted of flattening out my breast, so he pushed it with one hand and worked the ultrasound wand with the other. He needed the assistant to take the pictures with the machine. I was watching the screen intensely and realized there really **was** something there! I could see the spot in question. I asked if what I saw was the suspicious area, and was told yes. The assistant stated I seemed quite calm about all this, and I told her, "God is in control." She dropped her jaw but quickly recovered. The technician smiled. I had been so sure nothing would show up; now how was I to react? This was getting more complex. After the ultrasound was over, the technician walked me out, as the hospital is a maze, and on the walk mentioned my faith was obvious. He then stated he was a Christian. God even had a hand in who was to do my ultrasound.

After the radiologist read the ultrasound, my doctor called me again! This was not good; doctors don't call patients this often. Seems the radiologist didn't like what he saw on the ultrasound anymore than he did the mammogram. So then I had to make an appointment with a surgeon for a biopsy[7].

Even the word sounded ominous. I called the surgeon's office to schedule an appointment but his schedule and mine would not mesh. It was early August and I had a Pastor and Christian Worker's conference the next week that I was not willing to miss. The following week, I had to be in Evansville, Indiana for a seminar. I would not miss this class either. The doctor was going on vacation the third week in August, so we finally set a date for the last week of the month. I felt God was in control, so I could safely attend these events and wait. I still expected it to be no big deal.

"And we know that God causes all things to work together for good to those who love God, to those who are called according to His purpose." (Romans 8:28.)

The day of my appointment with the surgeon, I was a little nervous. The reality of there being something in me that did not belong was starting to sink in. When I met the doctor, he immediately put me at ease. He reminded me of a television doctor, Dr. Marcus

Welby, who had a great bedside manner. This doctor even looked like a thinner version of Dr. Welby. He explained to me that I probably had a papiloma[8], which was normal. The issue was that sometimes they can turn cancerous. So he recommended that we not do a needle biopsy[9] but rather do a wide excision biopsy[10] and remove the entire milk duct where the papiloma was located. What this would do- is if it was a cancer starting, we would remove it all still encased in the milk duct and the problem would be gone. If it was not a cancer starting, we still would not have any further problems, so it was a win-win situation. I agreed and we set the date for the day after Labor Day.

The surgery went off without a hitch and I came through with flying colors. There was some tenderness and the incision was much bigger than I anticipated, but overall, I felt pretty good and was not complaining. I was sure the issue was now over and I could heal and get on with my life. The doctor seemed to think the same thing and told us as much. I had to return for a surgical follow-up on the 14th of September. We were so sure it was nothing; I went to this appointment alone.

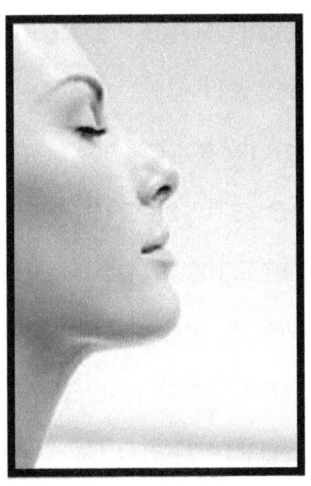

<u>Routine isn't so</u>
<u>Routine anymore...</u>

The doctor checked out my incision, we talked about how I was feeling, everything was progressing fine. Then he got a solemn look on his face and said "Everything looks good here, but your report isn't so good." My heart leapt into my throat and I looked up at him like I didn't hear him. I asked what he meant. He said, "It is intraductal carcinoma." [11] My brain went 'intraductal carcinoma, intraductal carcinoma, carcinoma, carcinoma means cancer. That means I have cancer.' I just looked at him unbelievingly for a few seconds until the reality sank in. He just sat there watching me.

The human brain is marvelous. Sometimes it seems to have a life of its own. After the reality sank in, my brain seemed to decide to ship me off somewhere and bring out only the medical social worker. Kaye, the cancer patient was out to lunch, but the social worker had a LOT of questions. When I started asking them, the doctor seemed stunned. He said I would not remember most of what he was telling me and wouldn't I like to wait and come back with my husband. I said, "Maybe later with Joe, but now I have questions and need answers." I wanted to know what stage[12] the cancer was at, what did the margins[13] show, I wanted to know best and worse case scenarios and I wanted a copy of my pathology report. [14] I knew I had research to do, and I needed the correct spelling of all those complex words to do it.

I was fine until the doctor patted me on the shoulder. That brought Kaye, the patient back and I started to cry. He was concerned about me being alone and driving (I live 20 miles from his office) but I said I could handle it. I knew God was with me. Hebrews 13:5 assures us; "I will never desert you, nor will I ever forsake you." I held on to that, but little did I realize how much of the driving God would have to do. As I drove I railed, I sobbed, I questioned, I wanted to stomp my feet and have a temper tantrum. And I pleaded with God, as I was concerned how my husband would handle this news.

Once I arrived home I had time to think, as my husband was not yet there. I wanted to tell him and was getting angry he wasn't there. James 1:19 came to mind: *"This you know, my beloved brethren. But let everyone be quick to hear, slow to speak and slow to anger"* followed by Ephesians 4:26: *"Be angry, and yet do not sin; do not let the sun go down on your anger."* Then I remembered he thought it was routine too, just like I had a few hours ago. When Joe arrived I barely had time to tell him before we had to leave to go to the airport. His daughter and her family were flying in for a week. We have an annual corn roast (big family get together of my husband's family) and it was in three days. Joe responded with "you are getting them cut off aren't you?" I had to explain I didn't know yet as I didn't have enough information to make any decision, but that was the way I was leaning.

All I wanted to do was research this diagnosis and try to decide what was happening to me. But I couldn't. I had a house full of people, a party going on, a 16 month old - who didn't understand why Gramma wouldn't/couldn't pick him up (as I was still recovering from the biopsy surgery) and my emotions were in a tale spin. There was no rhyme or reason to what was happening in my life. Everything seemed to go on as usual but nothing was normal anymore. Boy, could I see where I had counseled previous patients so inadequately since I did not understand what they were feeling. I wanted to shout at everyone, "Don't you see life has changed? It will never be the same again?" But I didn't. I acted like it was all okay and I held fast to the fact that God was in control.

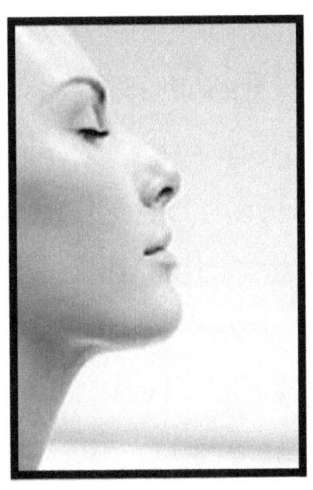

So Much Information – So Few Choices

Every spare minute I had I was on the internet. I read more about intraductal carcinoma than I thought possible. What I found only solidified my decision to have a double mastectomy[15]. What I couldn't figure out and needed answers to was how can it be only in the milk ducts and not have clear margins? Did I need lymph nodes[16] taken out? No where could I find the answers, I just kept getting more questions. Plus, everyone had an opinion of what I should do. I couldn't believe how many women were coming out of the woodwork who were breast cancer survivors. Friends I had no idea had cancer, were saying, "I have seven years or nine years or more under my belt." "I chose a mastectomy and reconstructive surgery." "I had only a lumpectomy", etc. I didn't want to talk to all these women, and then I did want to. More confusion, what should I do?

I found the information on the web sites [17], especially the medical sites, helpful. I could read and absorb only as much as I wanted to or was able to at one time. I preferred emails to talking, as I could turn it off if I couldn't deal with it. But I gathered enough information to know I wanted all breast tissue off my body. I had multi-focal[18] intraductal carcinoma and it was trying to kill me. It was found early[19] and if the entire breast was gone, there was no where else it could show up. The only thing I was not sure about was if lymph nodes needed to be removed[20]. Could the cancer have spread to the lymph system[21]? Many people were telling me I had to have nodes removed to make sure. Yet removing lymph nodes added all kinds of complications. [22] If I had any removed I only wanted a sentinel node[23] removed to check first.

On Monday I called the surgeon, who had done the initial biopsy, and scheduled an appointment to ask all my questions. After the research I had done, I had lots of questions. My cancer was apparently a stage zero or one, but the recommended treatment was total mastectomy.[24] This was not going to go away easily. The appointment was for Thursday. A week after I had found out it was cancer. A day after the kids flew home. Had it only been a week?

The doctor was great in answering many of our questions, but he didn't have the answers I wanted. He called a double mastectomy cruel and unusual to a woman and would not do one. He also talked about the length of time in surgery and the risks involved.[25] He talked about many, if not all, the lymph nodes being removed if a mastectomy was done. This is a radical mastectomy.[26] He also didn't want to discuss sentinel node biopsies, and said he was old school. I saw Joe wavering on the double mastectomy and getting stressed. This is my body, my life, me, we are talking about. Why don't I feel like I have any say in what happens? God help me to know what to do...

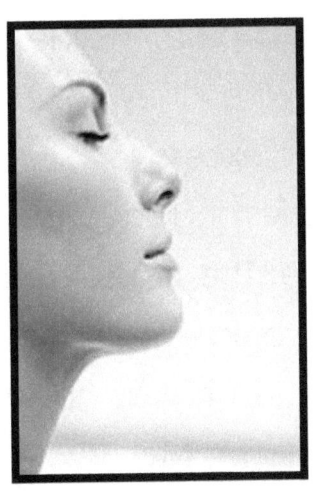

Why doesn't anyone want to listen?

As a social worker, I was amazed at the way the medical professionals were making choices for me without listening to me. I have worked in the medical field for years and often had patients tell me how helpless they felt. I thought they were talking about having the illnesses they had. Now, I'm not so sure. The doctor was not hearing me when I spoke. He was telling me I could not do what I wanted to do. The idea of removing a whole breast when they could remove only part of it seemed excessive to him. The idea of repeated surgeries and uncertainties sounded ridiculous to me. The first surgeon could not imagine that I would even consider a double mastectomy when it was not needed. Not needed for whom? My psychological well being needed this disease gone! Then when I found a doctor who would even discuss it, the second question was, "What does your husband say?" I agree my husband had a role here, and his support was important, but it was still my body. If this was any other cancerous appendage, they would cut it off, but they didn't want to remove the whole breast. This just didn't make sense to me. So I started asking all sorts of questions of all kinds of people.

When I spoke to other cancer victims who had mastectomies, most had had reconstructive surgery. [27] Of those with the reconstructive surgery, about 75% regretted having the implants. [28] When asked why they did it, they said for their husbands. Yet, when questioned further, they made the decision without discussing it with their spouses. The husbands did not care, they wanted their wives healthy. Of these same women, many were having continuing health problems related to the implants. [29]

I spoke with nurses, who cared for and were cancer victims themselves. All who chose to have mastectomies had no regrets. Those who had lumpectomies were fearful every time they felt anything out of the ordinary and were always concerned the cancer was coming back. One nurse admitted her sister had a double mastectomy and never regretted it. She has gone on and is living a full life. She did not have implants either. Yet, this same nurse had breast cancer and opted for a lumpectomy, chemo and radiation. She says she regrets her decision daily. She fears the cancer will return and lives with that fear daily. Her mother had died of breast cancer as well.

She has a third sister, who is still cancer free but is contemplating a double mastectomy as a preventative measure. This nurse looked around to make sure no one was in earshot and told me I had made the right decision. She then looked at Joe and said she was glad he was supportive. This was the last straw, so I had to ask her if other husband's were not supportive. She seemed shocked and said, "Oh yes, we have had husbands leave their wives over this." I was stunned!

No wonder the doctors try so hard to convince women to conserve their breasts. Has our society gotten so skewed that a woman cannot be a woman without breasts? Is a woman's value to herself or others based on physical beauty or proportions? I thought of 1 Peter 3:3-4, which tells us: "let not your adornment be *merely* external--braiding the hair, and wearing gold jewelry, or putting on dresses; but *let it be* the hidden person of the heart, with the imperishable quality of a gentle and quiet spirit, which is precious in the sight of

God." Yet, everything I was being told, was in direct opposition to what Peter said. This was an eye-opener for me. This philosophy was so unfair and was keeping women from being given all the information and options they need to make intelligent decisions; decisions that could save their lives. I remember my mother opting for a lumpectomy as she wanted to still feel like a woman. I didn't understand her thoughts then and only now am beginning too.

Prior to my bilateral mastectomy I was well endowed. I guess part of who I was, was in being large breasted, but I was also large all-over. I had long ago gotten over the hour-glass figure mentality and had accepted me as I was. Now I was going to lose one of the features society saw as a positive... How would I handle that? I needed to trust God and remember He was in control.

5

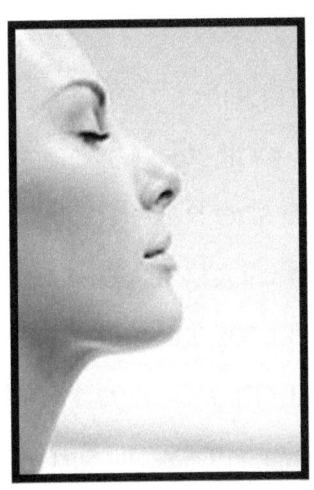

This is My Body, My Life, Me

I was more mixed up after leaving the doctor's than before I got there. Why was everything so complex? I didn't want to face one breast off and one on. I didn't want the chance of cancer coming back and I certainly didn't want to face two different surgeries.

As for the lymph node removal, that was a definite no. So since I knew what I wanted and the doctor definitely disagreed, what move did I make next? I started praying in earnest. About ten that night a friend called and said she just had to call. G never calls that late, but as we talked she helped put so much into perspective I felt God was behind the call. The next day I called my primary care physician. She only works until noon on Fridays and the chance of getting in was slim at best, but I called anyway. I was told there was an 11:30 appointment and I could have it. So off I went to see her. I told her what was happening and all the research I had done so far. I explained I had spoken to many cancer victims, and all said male doctors did not want to do double mastectomies. I also knew of two female doctors who would, but I didn't want to go that far from home; anyway I would need a referral from her to even see them. After many tears and questions Dr. K stated she knew a female plastic surgeon and would I like her to contact Dr. C and get an opinion? I said, "Yes" so she called her. Dr. C called back and after an extended conversation, when Dr. K got off the phone I had an appointment with the surgeon, a date for surgery and a pre-surgical physical scheduled. An appointment with the oncologist was pending; but Dr. K said she thought it might have to be after the surgery as he was booked solid in October, and October was also a month full of Jewish holidays. Since the oncologist was Jewish she doubted I would get in anytime that month. She would follow up on that appointment though and would let me know. As I left I looked back and requested she ask for the appointment to be the 11th as I had to be in Marquette that day anyway. She looked at me like I was not listening and reminded me I probably couldn't even get in anytime in October. I smiled and said, "God has been in control of every move so far and He is the God of Abraham, Isaac and Jacob, the God of the Jews, as well as the Christians; so just ask, please." Acts 3:13 states: *"The God of Abraham, Isaac, and Jacob, the God of our* fathers, has glorified His servant Jesus." She was shaking her head as I left.

When I arrived home, there was a message on my answering machine stating I had an appointment with the oncologist on the 11th at noon. My doctor's voice sounded stunned. I thought "Thanks God, you are even allowing me to witness through this." This was just another time God would show His hand so obviously at work in this continuing saga.

At the consultation with Dr. C, the plastic surgeon, she decided she was not the doctor to do the surgery, that I needed a general surgeon who would take closer margins. I said, "Only if he will do the double!" I was getting upset thinking, "here I go again." But, Dr. C said, "There are five general surgeons in this office, if the first one says no, I'll go to the next until I find one who will." She left the room only to return a couple minutes later. She explained there was only one surgeon in the office right then and he was looking over my chart. I started to ask a question, and she

said, "No, wait. Dr. R will be in, in a minute."
Now I was stunned. This clinic has a waiting list
to even get in of up to four months. My doctor
had pulled strings so I could see Dr. C. Now we
were switching doctors in mid-stream and I
was seeing the second doctor the same day!
Dr. R came in and we had a brief consultation.
He agreed to do the surgery and said we had
to select a date. I explained, "I thought the
surgery was already scheduled for the 24th
and I have a lot of prayer support set up for
that date. Was there any way we could keep
it?" Psalms 34:17 assures us: "*The righteous* cry
and the LORD hears, And delivers them out
of all their troubles." James 5:15-16 also tells
us: "*... the prayer offered in faith will restore
the one who is sick, and the Lord will raise
him up, and if he has committed sins, they
will be forgiven him. Therefore, confess your
sins to one another, and pray for one another,
so that you may be healed. The effective
prayer of a righteous man can accomplish
much.*" He looked at a calendar and smiled.

He said, "I do surgery on that day, so yes we'll keep it." Then he looked at his watch, told me I did not need to have the pre-surgical physical but I did need to go now in order to make my appointment with the oncologist and that he would call him before I got there. Anyone dealing with the medical field knows this is not the normal situation. Everything was falling into place like a well-oiled machine. My eleven o'clock appointment had turned into two appointments and I still made it to the one scheduled at noon. The only explanation was God was in control!

The next stop was the oncologist's office. There he gave me all sorts of options and choices. When he was done explaining everything, I finally convinced him (no one wanted to believe me) that I wanted a double mastectomy. When he was convinced I would not change my mind, he smiled. He then told me unless they found something unexpected he would not need to see me again. I said, "What about the radiation and chemo you were just talking about?" He assured me with the choice I made, I would leave the hospital cancer free and he did not need to see me again. The only explanation I could find was God was in control!

I did learn during this time how important it was to me to have some say in what was happening to me. I understood God was in control of the big picture, but I needed some control in the decisions being made about my care. I could not let the doctors make all the decisions. As a social worker, I realized how important it was for the patient to be involved in the decision making process.

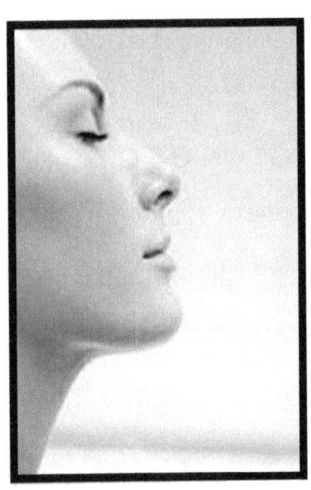

On top of everything else, there is Insurance!

S o now, I had someone listening but there was another problem. The insurance was getting into the decision making. If everyone has to go through this, the system needs to be fixed. Just when someone is feeling the most vulnerable, the insurance steps in and says, "No, you still can't make the decisions about your own body, we will." I could not believe now that the doctors were willing to do a double mastectomy, the insurance might nix it. The second breast did not test positive for cancer, so it is not necessary to remove it. It was an elective surgery and not covered. Who were they kidding? About this time, I was getting downright indignant. Being a Christian, I knew God was in control, but I sure felt Satan was trying hard to trip me up. 1 Peter 5:8 says: *"Be of sober spirit, be on the alert. Your adversary, the devil, prowls about like a roaring lion, seeking someone to devour."* So I started looking at options again. I found I could still have the double, but the insurance might only pay for the single. This would mean a major cost to me, but the insurance would have to cover the operating room, the anesthetic, etc. I just didn't think that was right, nor fair. I also thought about all the other women who would make a decision based on this information. How many would opt for removal of one, and reconstructive surgery because it was paid for. Yet, they would live with the fear of the cancer showing up in the second breast every day thereafter.

I started calling anyone I could think of.

Doctors said there was nothing they could do, so I turned to the lawyers. The consensus was it might take some time, and lots of appeals, but eventually the insurance would pay, especially with my family's history of cancer and mom dying of breast cancer. One lawyer even offered to take the case, if it became a case, pro bono. I decided to simply go ahead and see what would happen. Of course, I did call in prayer support for the cost to be covered by the insurance, and remembered God was in control. Luke 1:10 reminded me: " *And the whole multitude of the people were in prayer outside at the hour of the incense offering.*"

As a patient I was getting mad and frustrated that insurance could control what would happen to me. This was my life we were talking about not what choice of meat to have for dinner. It seemed ridiculous to me that money played a role and the insurance would decide on something trying to kill me. As a social worker I was flabber-gasted to think of all the patients who endured extra stress because of our medical insurance field's uncompassionate attitude. I could picture so many times in the past that I did not recognize where my clients true concerns were coming from. I did not realize the way the insurance companies made decisions was hampering the medical field personnel, not assisting them. Not only are the patients hands tied, their minds are bombarded with unnecessary choices related to insurance and money when they should be concentrating on getting well. How many patients make a bad choice to save money, or because they could not afford another choice? The doctor's hands are also tied. The insurance not only tells them they will not get paid for certain diagnostic or medical procedures but the insurance also tells them what they can or cannot do. The insurance companies are making medical decisions based on business practices without the medical knowledge necessary to make these assessments.

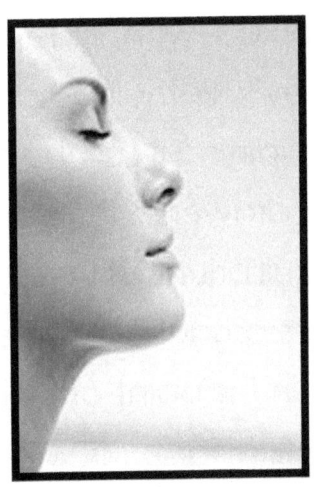

An Uncertain Path

*P*roverbs 3:6 says: "*In all your ways acknowledge Him, and He will make your paths straight.*" I sure was glad to know God was directing my path because I was not certain about it. I had some real fears and concerns and yet I tried so hard to be strong for everyone else around me. One concern I had was how this would affect my balance. Every time I asked this question, I was greeted with laughter. No one believed I was serious.

Yet, I have worked with elderly men who complained they lose their balance so much easier, even explaining it as "their chests have fallen into their drawers." In actuality a man does lose his equilibrium as he ages. His chest does fall and his stomach becomes a paunch, causing a shift in his point of balance. This is a proven scientific fact, so why wouldn't a woman who loses her breasts have the same problem, especially if the breasts are large? It seemed as if no one would take me seriously though.

I knew the choice I had made was the only one I could make but that did not make it any easier. I had to wonder how would I respond to no breasts after having large breasts since I was a pre-teen. What clothes would I be able to wear? How soon could I have my prosthetics[30], so I could go out? I did have some reservations about what I would be able to do after surgery. Would my arms work? What about strength? I was still recovering from knee surgery and depended on my arm strength to compensate for my weakened knee. With all these doubts, I was uncannily calm. I think I finally understood what Jesus meant when he said, *"Peace I leave with you; My peace I give to you; not as the world gives, do I give to you. Let not your heart be troubled, nor let it be fearful.* (John 14:27) The outcome was not what was important. Knowing God was and is in Control and this was a witnessing opportunity was what I focused on. This allowed me to head into surgery without fear; something I had never done before.

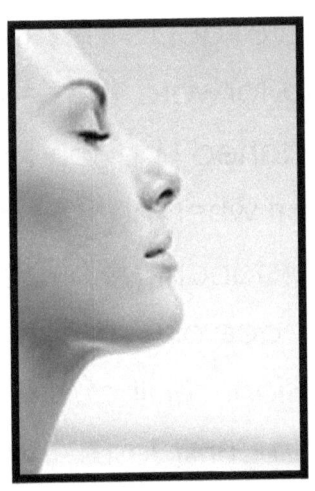

The Problem is
the Tunnel

Even though I knew God was in control and I had made the right choice, I still had to go through the surgery. I do not like surgery and this would be my third one in under a year. [31] I didn't have any choice, I had to do this. I had to face the fears, the unknown and go through that tunnel. I wasn't worried about death, but I sure didn't like the unknown of the tunnel, and what they (the pathologists) might find[32] before I got to the other side. I also was not looking forward to the recovery. As the day approached I began to understand what Paul meant when he said a peace that passes all understanding. Philippians 4:7 tells this: *"And the peace of God, which surpasses all comprehension, shall guard your hearts and your minds in Christ Jesus."* I was at peace. I was not worried, I was not scared and I didn't even care if I didn't make it through surgery. I knew if I didn't I would be in a much better place. I held on to Jesus' promise in Luke 23:43: *"And He said to him, "Truly I say to you, today you shall be with Me in Paradise."* I knew God was in control! My biggest fear was my husband and how he was dealing with all of this. God even handled that.

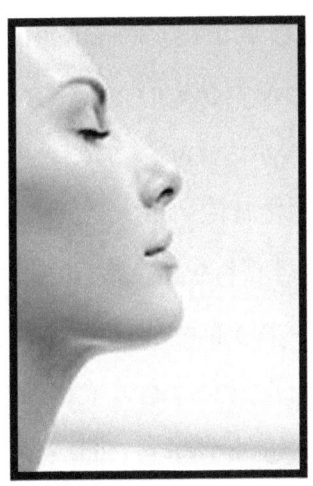

God Knew who Joe would need

Back in 2001, my husband and I opened a ministry. I wanted this ministry to be incorporated to protect the board members and to be able to be a tax exempt organization as it developed. So I worked closely with an attorney, to do the incorporation aspect of the ministry. Once it was incorporated, we decided to go ahead and apply for the tax exempt status. We worked with an acquaintance of Joe's, a

CPA who worked with non-profit corporations. Little did we know how important a role these two would play with my cancer ordeal.

When the attorney found out about my cancer he asked if he could tell his brother-in-law, a minister, who lived in a small town near the hospital I would be having surgery in. I said, "Of course" as I would take all the prayers I could get. Pastor R then contacted me via email and we kept in touch up until my surgery date. He promised he would be at the hospital before I went in and he was true to his word, arriving about 6:00 a.m. He prayed with both of us and stayed with Joe once I went into surgery. He had told me he had a hectic schedule and would try to come back, but I assured him my priority was for him to be with Joe while I was in surgery and thanked him for being there, even if he didn't make it back afterwards.

Another surprise of how much God was in control well before my diagnosis, was the selection of our CPA. When he found out about my ordeal, he invited Joe to stay with him and his wife while I was in the hospital. They then extended the invitation to both of us for the evening before surgery. We live 2 ½ hours from the hospital, they live 15 minutes away. We took them up on this offer and we had dinner, fellowship and a place to stay closer to the hospital. Their fellowship and prayers helped me deal with a difficult evening.

On the day of my surgery, not only did Pastor R arrive and stay with Joe but our CPA did as well. The three of them had quite an enjoyable time as Joe tells it and were surprised when the doctor came and told them I was in recovery. Joe said his reaction was "Already?" God's hand was involved not only with our ministry, but in placing these people into our lives so they would be there when we needed them the most. Deuteromony 31:8 assures us: *"And the LORD is the one who goes ahead of you; He will be with you. He will not fail you or forsake you. Do not fear, or be dismayed."* God was again in control even setting things and people in place, years ahead of time.

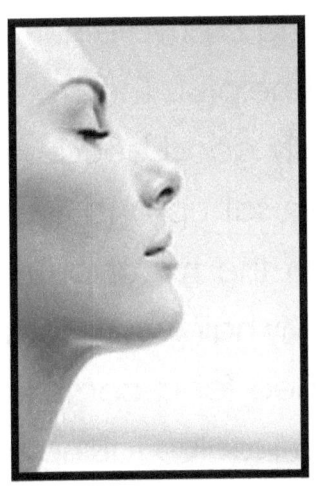

Coming Out of the Tunnel

When I woke up, I was already in my room. I didn't remember going into surgery, being in recovery or anything. In the previous two surgeries I had had that year, I remembered the operating room and talking with the nurses in recovery, so I was rather surprised to find myself already in my room. Joe was there as well as a nurse. It seems I had a student nurse assigned to me, so I felt really privileged. It was almost like having a private nurse. She was so enjoyable and helpful. The medication must have been really good because I was not in any pain. I even sat up and ate some lunch. Then I looked in the mirror on my table and thought, yipes! My hair was a disaster. Not even thinking I reached for a comb and combed it. Only later did I realize raising my arms over my head hurt. When I tried to do the same thing the next day my incisions pulled. Guess I probably shouldn't have been doing that the first day either. The cleaning lady came into my room about supper time (Joe had gone to eat) and we got talking. She could not believe I had only had surgery that morning, as I looked "too good" according to her. I just laughed. I think it was all the prayer support. I could tangibly feel the prayers. I even got up that evening (I had to use the facility as bed pans and I don't get along) and was pleasantly surprised to realize I did not feel like falling over backwards. Yes, I really WAS concerned about that. It was at this point some of the comedian in me, was born.

I had surgery on Monday morning and was released from the hospital on Wednesday morning. On Tuesday my surgeon had told me he wouldn't be in Wednesday until the afternoon, so when he showed up about 7:00 a.m. I was totally surprised. When he released me I was even more astonished, as I had told my husband to relax in the morning and not to come in until the afternoon. With the change of plans I had to find him so I could be discharged. I had to be gone before afternoon (again the insurance comes into play) to not be charged for an extra day. Once everything was done so I could leave, we left about 11:00. Needless to say, I got hungry enroute home. So I asked Joe to stop at a restaurant about 12:30. He just looked at me like I was crazy. He asked me, "You really feel like stopping at a restaurant? You have tubes[33], bandages and just got out of the hospital?" I replied, "I'm hungry. Yes, I can handle it, so stop please." We did. I guess I didn't think this was supposed to take that much out of me. I figured I should be able to just get on with life as usual.

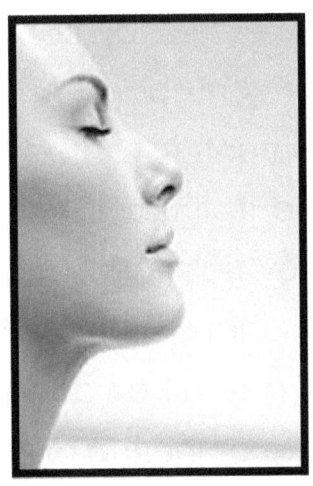

Life as Usual is not Familiar anymore

After arriving home from the hospital, I thought I could jump right back into doing everything, like some superwoman. Many people warned me it would take up to a year for the effects of the anesthesia to get out of my system, but I did not believe them. I had two surgeries earlier in the year and thought I was doing great, so this one wouldn't be much different. Boy was I wrong!

I got home on Wednesday from the hospital and rode with my husband on Friday to his doctor appointment. I wanted to say hi, as it was Dr. K. She just shook her head that I was out for a joy ride. On Sunday (six days since surgery) I attended Bible Study, in our basement. I did decline on attending church as the tubes were bothering me. On Monday we went back to Marquette and my tubes were removed. Freedom at last! My first question to the doctor was; "When can I drive?" He gave me the go ahead, so now there was no stopping me. Within the week I was driving to Sault Ste. Marie to go shopping. This is a town about 50 miles from my home. Not a good move. I did fine for a while and then the pain started. I still had to drive home. Maybe I am not such a superwoman after all!

During this time of recuperation I had to deal with emotional scars as well. To do this I became a comedian of sorts. I had done lots of research before surgery of what my options were. I found there was reconstructive surgery, prosthetics, or doing nothing. I opted for prosthetics and early on was using the fiber filled breasts[34]. There was only one problem, and it was major! These things were to light. They kept moving up my body and hitting my chin. This was not going to work! I had also found in my research that when breasts are reconstructed, if your nipple could not be salvaged, they could make you a new one.[35] To make it look more natural they tattooed[36] the color on. I just could not comprehend going into a tattoo parlor and asking for a nipple. Another option was stick on nipples.[37] This too sent me into gales of laughter. I could just visualize walking down the street and one popping off. Couldn't you imagine saying, "Excuse me Sir, but that is my nipple you just picked up off the sidewalk?" I couldn't! When I shared these comments with friends they all started laughing and told me having cancer and a bilateral mastectomy had turned me into quite a comedian. One close friend was quite insightful and said I was using laughter to hide behind. I explained; "not really it was just easier to laugh than to cry." Also being the social worker that I was, I wanted to put people at ease and being able to joke about it myself made others more comfortable around me. I had a psychologist friend tell me he was thrilled at the way I used laughter to help myself heal and to keep it up as laughter was good medicine. I had a strong Christian friend tell me he thought I was a great example of how a Christian should handle tough situations, and that helped more than anything. I had a pastor friend tell me he had questions he wanted to ask and was hesitant to do so, until he read my emails and I was so frank he felt he could be too. I had husbands thank me for helping them finally be able to talk with their wives about breast cancer, after talking with me. As a social worker and Christian I felt good I could put others at ease and help.

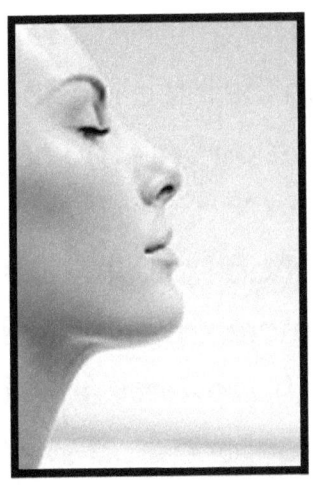

<u>*Will I ever be Me again?*</u>

This was getting to me! It was just too much. I figured I could have the surgery and just get on with my life. I have too much to do to have all these complications. I have gotten used to the breasts being gone, but not to the spare tire showing so much now. Before the breasts hid it from my view when I looked down and my clothes hung differently. Now all that shows is my stomach, and I don't like it. I just feel so rotten, why did I survive to just feel like this? Why do I feel so distraught? First the cancer, then the surgery, then the infection, then falling and getting a concussion[38] and hurting my knees[39]. Will it never end? God, you aren't supposed to give me more than I can handle, but I can't handle this anymore. 1 Corinthians 10:13 tells us: *"No temptation has overtaken you but such as is common to man; and God is faithful, who will not allow you to be tempted beyond what you are able, but with the temptation will provide the way of escape also, that you may be able to endure it."* I know you are in control, and in my weakness is your strength, but I need more help! 2 Corinthians 12:9-10 assured me: *"And He has said to me, "My grace is sufficient for you, for power is perfected in weakness." Most gladly, therefore, I will rather boast about my weaknesses, that the power of Christ may dwell in me. Therefore I am well content with weaknesses, with insults, with distresses, with persecutions, with difficulties, for Christ's sake; for when I am weak, then I am strong."* This is all well and good, but the social worker in me is getting concerned about me the patient.[40] I am not suicidal, but I have no will to live. I felt like Elijah, in 1Kings 19:4 when he said: *"But he himself went a day's journey into the wilderness, and came and sat down under a juniper tree; and he requested for himself that he might die, and said, "It is enough; now, O LORD, take my life. Life just isn't worth all this pain."* Even remembering Paul and what he said in 2 Corinthians 12:7-8: is not helping me. Paul said *"... for this reason, to keep me from exalting myself, there was given me a thorn in the flesh, a messenger of Satan to buffet me-- to keep me from exalting myself! Concerning this I entreated the Lord three times that it might depart from me."* If Paul and Elijah went through this, why not me? But knowing this, doesn't change the fact; I am still having a hard time acting like a comedian and laughing. I remind myself of a clown with a painted smile who is crying underneath and no one knows it. I think depression[41] has set in...

Since I think of myself as a Biblical counselor

and I know a doctor who treats himself has an uncooperative patient, I need a different Biblical Counselor. So, I called my mentor and asked for help. Exodus 18:19 says *"Now listen to me: I shall give you counsel, and God be with you."* He advised me, I needed to get back into my studies even if I only answered one question or wrote one paragraph a day. I still needed to do at least that and to do it whether I felt like it or not. I also needed to get back into counseling others. He laughingly told me he wasn't telling me anything I didn't already know, it was just I was hearing it differently. So I attempted doing that. I worked at school but my heart wasn't in it. I counseled using God's word and letting the Holy Spirit guide, but I didn't let Him guide me. I couldn't shake the despair I felt. I didn't feel like me and was afraid I might never get me back.

I had been doctoring for arthritis in my knee and had surgery on it prior to being diagnosed with cancer. It was again flaring up and the pain was excruciating on top of the depression. I cried out to God numerous times to please let me come home. Jonah 4:3 tells us: *"Therefore now, O LORD, please take my life from me, for death is better to me than life."* It felt like he just ignored me. As a Biblical counselor I remembered Christ's words on the cross, in Matthew 27:46, which says: *"About the ninth hour Jesus cried out with a loud voice, saying,... "My God, My God, why hast thou forsaken Me?"* I began to understand the desperation of that statement. I think it is included in the Bible to help us when we feel God has forsaken us, and to remind us that He never forsakes us, even when we feel that He has. Psalms 73:23-24 says: *"Nevertheless I am continually with Thee; Thou hast taken hold of my right hand. With Thy counsel Thou wilt guide me, And afterward receive me to glory."*

In August I had shots in my knee which helped ease the pain, and I thanked God for the help. 2 Corinthians 4:15 (NIV)says: *"All this is for your benefit, so that the grace that* is reaching more and more people may cause thanksgiving to overflow to the glory of God." As the summer ended, I started doing somewhat better physically, but emotionally I was a wreck. Nothing interested me. So I again called on my mentor and cried out for help. This time he gave me an example that helped to put things in focus. I realized I was not in the will of God and needed to make some changes. That was why I was unhappy and discouraged. Psalms 143:10 explains: *"Teach me to do Thy will, For Thou art my God; Let Thy good Spirit lead me on level ground."* I changed my major in school and for the first time in over a year was excited about something again. As the year anniversary of my surgery approached I found I was feeling better not only physically but emotionally and spiritually. I was finally on the road to recovery. They weren't kidding when they said the effects would last a year.

Each day is a blessing from God and I am reminded of that often. I thank Him daily that my cancer was found and cured. I am reminiscent of the blessing it took for that to occur every morning when I wake up. I hope now to be able to say and mean as Paul did in Philippians 1:21; *"For to me, to live is Christ, and to die is gain."* I do not need to be me; I need to be Christ in me! Looking back this has been the most difficult year of my life and yet I would not change it. I would do it all over again, just because of what I learned and of how close it has brought me to my Lord. And Yes, GOD **IS** IN CONTROL!

End Notes/Explanations:

1. **Lumpectomy.** A surgical procedure that removes the breast lump or suspicious tissue... and some surrounding tissue as well. http://www.dcis.info/treatment-options.html

2. **Radiation.** The use of radiology, a branch of medicine concerned with the use of radiant energy (as x-rays and radium) in the diagnosis and treatment of disease. (Merriam-Webster, 599)

3. **Stress effects health.** Mind-body interaction. Social and psychological stress can trigger or aggravate a wide variety of diseases... Most people, on the basis or either intuition or personal experience, believe that emotional stress can precipitate or alter the course of even major physical diseases... Psychological factors can also indirectly influence a disease's course. (Berkow, 390)

4. **Mammogram**. The picture that is the result of mammography (a test that uses low-level x-rays to find abnormal areas in the breast) is one of the best ways to detect breast cancer early. (Berkow, 1099)

5. **Radiologist.** A physician specializing in the use of radiant energy for diagnostic and therapeutic purposes. (Merriam-Webster, 600)

6. **Ultra-sound**. The diagnostic or therapeutic use of ultra-sound and esp. a technique involving the formation of a two dimensional image used for the examination and measurement of internal body structures and the detection of bodily abnormalities. (Webster, 740)

7. **Biopsy**. The removal and examination of tissue, cells, or fluids from the living body. (Webster, 76)

8. A **papiloma** is a benign tumor, as a polyp or wart, of the skin or mucous membrane,

consisting of a group of thickened, enlarged papillae. Such a tumor caused by a virus.

9. **A needle biopsy** is a procedure whereby a doctor inserts a needle attached to a syringe to extract a section of tissue/cells where a lump has been found to determine if it is cancerous or benign. This procedure examines the lump but does not examine surrounding tissue (Berkow, 1101)

10. **Wide excision biopsy.** A form of breast conserving surgery, consisting of removal of the tumor and somewhat more surrounding normal tissue. (Berkow, 1103)

11. **Intraductal Cacinoma** is a name used to describe a form of breast cancer. It is also known as ductal carcinoma in situ or DCIS. Ductal carcinoma in situ is a precancerous condition characterized by the clonal proliferation of malignant-looking cells in the lining of a breast duct without evidence of spread outside the duct to other tissues

in the breast. DCIS is clearly the precursor of invasive breast cancer. This is evident from the sharing of clonal chromosome changes by DCIS and adjacent invasive cancers. www.medterms.com/script/main/art.asp?articlekey=31789

12. **Staging** of cancer is base on the size of the tumor, whether lymph nodes are involved, and whether the cancer has spread beyond the breast. www.breastcancer.org/pathology_intro.html

    NOTE: With DCIS, size has no impact on stage – this is unlike invasive breast cancer where size and stage are related. DCIS is always a stage 0, but it can be any size and be located in any number of areas inside the breast.
    www.breastcancer.org/dcis_extent_affects.html

13. **Margin** – is the term used to describe the area affected by the cancer. When they remove the breast tissue in a biopsy, the

tissue is examined to see how close to the edge the cancer is. If it goes all the way to the edge there is no clear margin and is called positive. A negative margin is am area free of cancer cells. Most pathologists agree that a margin of at least two millimeters is best. The wider the margin, the lower the risk of the cancer coming back. A positive margin requires additional treatment as the cancer is still there. http://www.breastcancer.org/dcis_extent_affects.html

14. **Pathology Report**- This is the report written by the pathologist to explain what was found after examining the excised tissue. It includes identifying information about the patient, a description of the specimen examined including where if is from (i.e., for me it was the left breast); a short history of any breast abnormality and how it was found; the clinical diagnosis; the gross description describes the size, weight,

color, etc.; the microscopic description tells how it appears under the microscope and then the findings are summarized in the conclusion. http://www.breastcancer.org/pathology_intro.html

15. **Double or Bilateral Mastectomy.** Bilateral: of, relating to, or affecting the right and left sides of the body or the right and left members of paired organs. Mastectomy: Excision or amputation of a mammary gland [breast] and usu. associated tissue. (Webster, 73, 412)

16. **Lymph Nodes.** These are part of the lymphatic system that works in the body's immune defenses. The lymph nodes filter out foreign particles that get into the lymph – for example, cancer that have separated from a nearby cancerous growth. Lymph nodes also produce essential components of the immune system, including white blood cells that make antibodies to destroy to destroy foreign organisms. (Berkow, 147)

17. **Web sites.** The internet or World Wide Web is a source of information. Many of the websites used in researching my cancer are listed in the Bibliography.

18. **Multi-focal** Intraductal carcinoma means more than one area of DCIS in one quadrant. www.breastcancer.org/dcis_extent_affects.html

19. **Early Detection.** Early detection means finding the cancer while it is still in the early stages and easily treated. The more advanced the cancer the less successful the treatment options. Early detection is key to survival. "This year in America, more than 211,000 women will be diagnosed with breast cancer and 43,300 will die... In addition, 1,600 men will be diagnosed with breast cancer and 400 will die. If detected early, the five-year survival rate exceeds 95%. http://.www.thebreastcancersite.com/cgi-bin/WebObjects/CTDSites

20. **Lymph node removal**. Doctors evaluate lymph nodes when a cancer is diagnosed to determine if it has spread. This is why removal can be critical in cancer diagnosis and treatment. (Berkow, 147)

21. **Lymph System**. The immune system maintains its own system of circulation - the lymphatic vessels - which permeates every organ in the body except the brain... Along the lymphatic vessels are special areas – the lymph nodes, tonsils, bone marrow, spleen, liver, lungs, and intestines. (Berkow, 807)

22. **Lymph node removal complications**: Often if lymph nodes are removed a complication called lymphedema occurs. This is when excess fluid collects in the arms or legs. This condition can be persistent and interfere with activities of daily living. American Cancer Society. *Breast Cancer Dictionary.*

23. **Sentinel Node**: This is the lymph node closest to the cancer site. A sentinel node biopsy is a new procedure where blue dye and a radioactive tracer are injected into the tumor site at the time of surgery and the first (sentinel) node that picks up the dye is removed and biopsied. If the node is cancer-free, fewer nodes are removed. American Cancer Society. *Breast Cancer Dictionary.*

24. **Total Mastectomy**: A simple, total mastectomy is a procedure in which the entire breast is removed but not the lymph nodes under the arm or the muscle tissue from beneath the breast. The nipple will be removed in this procedure, but much of the original skin of the breast may be preserved. www.dcis.info/treatment-options.html

25. **Surgical risks**: It's important to remember that the techniques used in breast cancer surgery have improved dramatically in recent years. But as you probably know,

any kind or surgery... involves risk. ... Some of the risks and complications associated with breast cancer surgery are: wound infections, and/or problems with wounds healing. Excessive bleeding, during or after breast cancer surgery is rare. If you are planning a more extensive surgery, such as a double mastectomy... you may consider donating blood before surgery. Another risk is any time you go under general anesthesia, you put yourself at some risk, although the risks, today are extremely low – around one death in 200,000 cases. The longer you are under anesthesia the higher the risk. Sometimes after surgery it may be harder than before for lymph fluid to drain from the arm. The can result in swelling, called lymphedema. http://www. breastcancer.org/tre_surg_fearrisks.html

26. **Radical Mastectomy**: A radical mastectomy is just that, **radical**. It includes removal of the entire breast, all underarm lymph

nodes, and chest wall muscles under the breast. Although it was common in the past, radical mastectomy is now rarely performed because modified radical mastectomy has proven to be just as effective and less disfiguring. Today radical mastectomy is recommended only when cancer has spread to the chest muscles under the breast. www.breastcancer.org/tre_surg_mastectomy.html

27. **Reconstructive surgery.** After a general surgeon removes a breast tumor and the surrounding breast tissue, a plastic surgeon may reconstruct the breast, using a silicone or saline implant or in a more complex operation, tissue taken from other parts of the woman's body, usually the abdomen. (Berkow, 1105)

28. **Breast Implants:** An artificial form used to restore the shape of a breast after surgery. American Cancer Society. *Breast Cancer Dictionary.*

29. **Health Problems related to implants**: Breast implant problems can range in severity from mild nuisances to life-threatening incidents... Breast implant problems such as capsular contracture, leakage, or even rupture may be possible. Often repeated surgeries are needed to repair the problems. www.ebreastaug.com/breast-implant/problems.html

30. **Prosthetics**: An artificial form, such as a breast prosthesis, that can be worn under the clothing after a mastectomy. American Cancer Society. *Breast Cancer Dictionary.*

31. **Third surgery.** My bilateral mastectomy was my third surgery in under a year. The first being April 7th to clean up my injured left knee. I had not recovered fully from this surgery when the cancer was found. The second surgery was the wide excision to remove the milk duct on September 7th. The third was the bilateral mastectomy on October 24th.

32. **Pathologist found a Surprise**: When I returned to the surgeon, for my post surgical check-up, he explained what the pathologists found in my breasts. There was a cancerous lump, hidden behind the nipple and was about ½ inch in size. This cancer did not show up in all the previous tests. He explained, had we not removed the entire breast this cancer would have been invasive in under a year.

33. **Drainage tubes.** After surgery there are tubes left in place to help your body drain the excess fluid and blood caused by the surgical procedure. I personally was discharged with two tubes in my chest, one on each side. These tubes were attached to small plastic bulbs that caught the fluid, and had to be emptied daily.

34. **Fiber filled**: The American Cancer Society sent me a nylon pocket-type prosthetic that could be filled with fiberfill stuffing. It was then inserted into your bra, similar

to falsies. The fiber fill was lightweight and would not stay in place.

35. **New nipple**: The nipple could be reconstructed at the same time the breast was. The decision to have this done is up to each patient. Reconstruction of the new nipple is usually done after the new breast has had time to settle and heal. Tissue for the new nipple and areola are taken from another part of your own body... The nipple from the breast that was removed would not be used as it could contain cancer cells. American Cancer Society. *Breast Reconstruction Following Mastectomy* pamphlet

36. **Tattoo.** Definition:) To puncture (the skin) with a needle and insert indelible colors so as to leave permanent marks or designs. (Agnes, 1466)

    Nipple tattooing:) If the shape of the nipple has not been created with surgery, a tattooing technique can be used to get the effect of a nipple and areola on the breast; this technique will not give the three-dimensional shape of a nipple but it can give a very good appearance... Nipple tattooing is usually done under local anesthetic... The procedure usually takes 30-40 minutes... Usually the tattooing procedure needs to be repeated to give the best results. http://www.cancerbackup.org. uk?Aboutcancer/Genetics/Risk-reducingbreastsurgery

37. **Stick-on Nipples**. Actually, these are nipple prosthetics or silicone stick-on nipples. They can be attached to the reconstructed breasts using special glue. These can be bought ready-made or can be custom made or can be an exact mould of the original nipple and areola. http://www. cancerbackup.org.uk?Aboutcancer/ Genetics/Risk-reducingbreastsurgery

38. **Concussion**. A condition resulting from the stunning, damaging, or shattering effects

of a hard blow; esp a jarring injury of the brain resulting in disturbances of cerebral function and sometimes marked by permanent damage. (Webster, 138)

39. **Reinjury to knees**. I had injured my knees previously, then had surgery on the left one in April. When I fell in January, I landed on my knees injuring both of them. Since they were already injured, rather than healing they became inflamed and kept getting worse, known as a downward spiral. To break the cycle, or spiral, cortisone shots were administered in both knees, on March 17th.

40. **Social Worker Concerns**. The mind-body interaction is a two-way street. Not only can psychological factors contribute to the onset or aggravation of a wide variety of physical disorders, but also physical diseases can affect a person's thinking or mood. People with life-threatening, recurring, or chronic physical disorders

commonly become depressed. Although depression under these circumstances may appear to be a normal reaction, the person's mental state still deserves attention. The depression may worsen the effects of the physical disease and add to the person's misery. (Berkow, 391)

41. **Depression.** A psychoneurotic or psychotic disorder marked esp. by sadness, inactivity, difficulty with thinking and concentration, a significant increase or decrease in appetite and time spent sleeping, feelings or rejection and hopelessness, and sometimes suicidal thoughts. (Webster, 172)

Scripture References Used throughout and for Comfort

📖 **James 4:15** Instead,, *you ought* to say, "If the Lord wills, we shall live and also do this or that."

📖 **Romans 8:28** And we know that God causes all things to work together for good to those who love God, to those who are called according to *His* purpose.

📖 **Hebrews 13:5** "I will never desert you, nor will I ever forsake you."

📖 **James 1:19** *This* you know, my beloved brethren. But let everyone be quick to hear, slow to speak *and* slow to anger;

📖 **Ephesians 4:26** Be angry, and *yet* do not sin; do not let the sun go down on your anger.

📖 **Peter 3:3-4** And let not your adornment be *merely* external--braiding the hair, and wearing gold jewelry, or putting on dresses; but *let it be* the hidden person of the heart, with the imperishable quality of a gentle and quiet spirit, which is precious in the sight of God.

📖 **Acts 3:13** "The God of Abraham, Isaac, and Jacob, the God of our fathers, has glorified His servant Jesus."

📖 **Psalms 34:17** *The righteous* cry and the LORD hears, And delivers them out of all their troubles.

📖 **James 5:15-16** … the prayer offered in faith will restore the one who is sick, and the Lord will raise him up, and if he has committed sins, they will be forgiven him. Therefore, confess your sins to one another, and pray for one another, so that you may be healed. The effective prayer of a righteous man can accomplish much.

📖 **1 Peter 5:8** Be of sober *spirit,* be on the alert. Your adversary, the devil, prowls about like a roaring lion, seeking someone to devour.

📖 **Luke 1:10** And the whole multitude of the people were in prayer outside at the hour of the incense offering.

📖 **Proverbs 3:6** In all your ways acknowledge Him, And He will make your paths straight.

📖 **John 14:27** "Peace I leave with you; My peace I give to you; not as the world gives, do I give to you. Let not your heart be troubled, nor let it be fearful.

📖 **Philippians 4:7** And the peace of God, which surpasses all comprehension, shall guard your hearts and your minds in Christ Jesus.

📖 **Luke 23:43** And He said to him, "Truly I say to you, today you shall be with Me in Paradise."

📖 **Deuteronomy 31:8** "And the LORD is the one who goes ahead of you; He will be with you. He will not fail you or forsake you. Do not fear, or be dismayed."

📖 **1 Corinthians 10:13** No temptation has overtaken you but such as is common to man; and God is faithful, who will not allow you to be tempted beyond what you are able, but with the temptation will provide the way of escape also, that you may be able to endure it.

📖 **2 Corinthians 12:9-10** And He has said to me, "My grace is sufficient for you, for power is perfected in weakness." Most gladly, therefore, I will rather boast about my weaknesses, that the power of Christ may dwell in me. Therefore I am well content with weaknesses, with insults, with distresses, with persecutions, with difficulties, for Christ's sake; for when I am weak, then I am strong.

📖 **1 Kings 19:4** But he himself went a day's journey into the wilderness, and came and sat down under a juniper tree; and he requested for himself that he might die, and said, "It is enough; now, O LORD, take my life

📖 **2 Corinthians 12:7-8** And because of the surpassing greatness of the revelations, for this reason, to keep me from exalting myself, there was given me a thorn in the flesh, a messenger of Satan to buffet me--to keep me from exalting myself! Concerning this I entreated the Lord three times that it might depart from me.

📖 **Exodus 18:19** "Now listen to me: I shall give you counsel, and God be with you.

📖 **Jonah 4:3** "Therefore now, O LORD, please take my life from me, for death is better to me than life."

📖 **Matthew 27:46** And about the ninth hour Jesus cried out with a loud voice, saying, "Eli, Eli, Lama Sabachthani?" that is, "My God, My God, why hast thou forsaken me?"

📖 **Psalms 73:23-24** Nevertheless I am continually with Thee; Thou hast taken hold of my right hand. With Thy counsel Thou wilt guide me, And afterward receive me to glory.

📖 **2 Corinthians 4:15** (New International Version) All this is for your benefit, so that the grace that is reaching more and more people may cause thanksgiving to overflow to the glory of God.

📖 **Psalms 143:10** Teach me to do Thy will, For Thou art my God; Let Thy good Spirit lead me on level ground.

📖 **Philippians 1:21 For to me, to live is Christ, and to die is gain.**

📖 **1 Peter 1:6-7** In this you greatly rejoice, even though now for a little while, if necessary, you have been distressed by various trials, that the proof of your faith, *being* more precious than gold which is perishable, even though tested by fire, may be found to result in praise and glory and honor at the revelation of Jesus Christ.

📖 **James 1:2-4** Consider it all joy, my brethren, when you encounter various trials, knowing that the testing of your faith produces endurance. And let endurance have *its* perfect result, that you may be perfect and complete, lacking in nothing.

📖 **Romans 8:18** For I consider that the sufferings of this present time are not worthy to be compared with the glory that is to be revealed to us.

📖 **2 Corinthians 1:3-4** Blessed be the God and Father of our Lord Jesus Christ, the Father of mercies and God of all comfort; who comforts us in all our affliction so that we may be able to comfort those who are in any affliction with the comfort with which we ourselves are comforted by God.

📖 **2 Corinthians 4:18** while we look not at the things which are seen, but at the things which are not seen; for the things which are seen are temporal, but the things which are not seen are eternal.

A What **TO DO and DO NOT DO** List for a **Patient**

DO:

1. Do find out what your patient rights and responsibilities are. If you do not understand, have someone explain them to you.

2. Do find a doctor you are comfortable with and trust.

3. Do look for professionals who specialize in your disease.

4. Do ask questions. If you do not understand all the implications of a treatment, ask questions, research it, do whatever is necessary for you to feel comfortable about the procedure. You do have the right to say no.

5. Do get a second opinion if you are uncomfortable.

6. Do keep a folder or notebook of all information, i.e., doctor appointments, procedures and results, research, questions, etc.

7. Do write out questions you have before your appointments. Be sure and ask early in the appointment.

8. Do take a note pad and pen with you to all exams and appointments.

9. Do request copies of all tests, procedures and reports. Keep in folder or notebook.

10. Do speak up if you feel you are being ran over or left out of the decision making process.

11. Do keep good records. Who you spoke to, what about, when, what did they say. This can be regarding procedures, treatment options, insurance coverage, etc.

12. Do talk with your insurance carrier to see what needs to be done. What do they cover, what documentation or pre-

authorization is needed. What will they not cover and can you appeal? Stay on top of this, but do not let them make the decisions on your life.

13. Do weigh all your options and what you can or cannot handle, i.e., having only one breast, additional surgeries, etc.

14. Do take the time you need to be alone or with your spouse to digest all the news.

15. Do pick someone to me your advocate, to attend appointments with you and help you to remember. This could be your spouse, family member, or friend.

16. Do keep some control, so you do not feel helpless. Talk with someone if you are feeling helpless and make them listen to you.

17. Do keep some routine in your life after a difficult diagnosis. Some normalcy.

18. Do be willing to work with your insurance, do not be afraid of them.

19. Do realize you can have a procedure even if your insurance does not cover it.

20. Do utilize The American Cancer Society for assistance.

21. Do keep in control of some decisions, it is important for your mental health to not feel helpless or useless.

22. If finances are a problem, do take time to drop a note to your creditors explaining. Most will work with you and this will reduce unwanted calls and stress.

23. Do realize stress affects your health and take appropriate actions.

24. Do keep your stress level as low as you can manage.

25. Do communicate with your spouse. Find out what he really thinks, feels, fears. Do not make decisions on what you think he wants, TALK and find out for sure. Find

out what he is really thinking about your disease and all treatment options.

26. Do talk with your children and family. They can imagine much worse than the reality. Be honest, but age appropriate.

27. Do realize who you are is not your breasts.

28. Do realize there is nothing you could have done to prevent getting this disease. It is not your fault.

29. Do ask for help, many people want to help but do not know how. You make them feel useful by asking.

30. Do accept help. Not only from those you ask, but those who offer.

31. Do remember you are still you, you are more than this disease. Live your life as much as you can.

32. Do realize you will not be completely healed from surgery when you return

home. You will probably still have tubes and open wounds, needing care

33. Do find time for yourself to relax. Read a book, pray, meditate. You need to stay strong to fight.

34. Do use prayer and tell your prayer warrior what specifically they can pray for.

35. Do eat healthy. Even when you don't feel like eating, you must. Use supplements if need be, but your body needs nourishment for battle.

36. Do exercise as tolerated.

37. Do realize there are others who have survived this. They are there if you want to talk with them. Remember the choice is yours.

38. Do realize you have a good chance of survival and of living a full life.

39. Do what you are comfortable with to deal with your diagnosis. I used joking, find what works for you.

40. Do talk with others if you are comfortable. If uncomfortable tell them that. They will take your lead.

41. Do admit you hurt and need help

42. Do give yourself time to heal, even from biopsies.

43. Do take the time you need. Do not rush into things to quickly.

44. Do concentrate on getting well, the rest can wait.

45. Do be aware of anesthesia effects.

46. Do recognize depression is not unusual and may even be part of the side effects of surgery, anesthesia, radiation or chemo.

47. Do cry out to God.

48. Do seek the counsel of others.

49. Do acknowledge your emotions, it's okay to get angry.

50. Do recognize the tangible feeling of prayer

may be gone. People may have been more attentive to you during your actual surgery, not your recovery.

51. Do keep your faith and trust God.

52. Do LAUGH when you can, and cry when you must. Both are okay and needed.

53. Do keep control. It is important to feel in control of your life, since the disease is controlling your body.

54. Do get regular mammograms and other routine exams.

DO NOT:

1. Do not assume your husband wants you to have breasts over health. Ask him!

2. Don't go to an appointment alone when you are unsure of the outcome.

3. Do not assume the doctor is always right. This is you and you have the ultimate say.

4. Do not accept anything you do not understand.

5. Do not be afraid. Ask questions until you feel comfortable.

6. Don't try to hide your feelings, fears, etc.

7. Do no get forced into any decision you are not comfortable with.

8. Do not get forced into anything you do not want to do.

9. Do not be rushed into making a decision. Time may be important but take a breath and look at all options before deciding. Taking an hour verses an immediate decision is usually not life threatening. Ask how much time you have to safely decide.

10. Do not accept a no from the insurance without appealing.

11. Don't have lots on your plate right after getting a diagnosis. Bow out of some things

or cancel if need be. Do only as much as you can handle, you will be dealing with a shock.

12. If you get a negative diagnosis, do not plan big or out-of-the ordinary events.

13. Do not make decisions based on money. Options are available.

14. Do not give up! Ever!

15. Do not try to be superwoman. Give yourself time to heal.

16. Do not make life effecting decisions based purely on appearance.

17. Do not take long trips, unless absolutely necessary.

18. Do not drive alone the first couple weeks after surgery. If you get tired or develop pain, you have help with you.

A What **TO DO** and **DO NOT DO** List for a **Social Worker**

DO:

1. Do listen to your client. If they say they feel helpless, explore how and why.

2. Do explain to them what their rights are, and that they do have say in their own treatment.

3. Do explain to them what the treatment consist of, pros and cons.

4. Do explain medical terminology that they find confusing.

5. Do encourage and assist with research.

6. Do help them to understand their insurance coverage.

7. Do help them understand the insurance jargon that they may find confusing.

8. Do help your client retain usefulness.

9. Do be an advocate for the client, with other professionals, insurance, creditors, etc.

10. Do help them with networking agencies to assist if financial needs are present.

11. Do explore options with them, as they are comfortable with to be sure they understand their options.

12. Do explain what they can actually expect of surgery, the length of stay and returning home with tubes, etc.

13. Do help them to understand relaxation techniques and how to handle and reduce stress.

14. Do encourage them to communicate with family. Assist if need be.

15. Do encourage them to live, not focus on their disease.

16. Do help to empower them.

17. Do encourage spiritual involvement to the level they are comfortable.

18. Do share your faith, and pray with client.

19. Do watch for sign and symptoms of depression.

DO NOT:

1. If they express fear, do not minimize it, encourage them to discuss it.

2. Do not dismiss any of their comments.

3. Do not assume they understand your explanation, have them explain back to you what they understood.

4. Do not offer advise where it is not wanted, i.e., marital, which decision they should make, etc.

5. Do not try to control them. They need control now more than ever.

6. Do not chastise the client for their behavior. They need encouragement not discipline, they are not children.

7. Do not treat them as if they were children.

8. Do not take over for the client, just assist.

9. Do not make any decisions for them. Advocate for their wishes not yours.

10. Do not judge them or their decisions. What is right for you may not be right for them.

BIBLIOGRAPHY

📖 Agnes, Michael, Editor in Chief, 2001, Webster's New World Dictionary 4th Edition. (Foster City, CA: IDG Books Worldwide, Inc.)

📖 Berkow, Robert M.D., Editor in Chief, 1997, Merck Manual of Medical Information Home Edition. (Whitehouse Station, NJ: Merck & Co., Inc.)

📖 Merriam-Webster. Webster's Medical Desk Dictionary. 1986 (Springfield, MA: Merriam-Webster, Inc.)

📖 Smith, Robert D., M.D., 2000, The Christian Counselor's Medical Desk Reference. (Stanley, NC, Timeless Texts)

📖 The American Cancer Society Pamphlets. (Oklahoma City,OK) Breast Reconstruction Following Mastectomy. 2001
Lymphedema. 2004.
The Breast Cancer Dictionary. 2003.

📖 The Holy Bible, New American Standard Bible (NASB), 1995. (La Habra, CA: The Lockman Foundation)

📖 The Holy Bible, New International Version (NIV) 1996. (Grand Rapids, MI: Zondervan)

WEBSITES:

(This list is not exhaustive, but lists the sites I personally found helpful)

➢ www.breastcancer.org Self explanatory.

➢ http://www.breastcancer.org/dcis extent_affects.html General information regarding breast cancer.

➢ http://www.breastcancer.org/ pathology_report.pdf This site is a guide to your pathology report. It contains a complete booklet (25 pages) that I found extremely beneficial.

➢ http://www.breastcancer.org/tre_surg fearrisks.html This site has good info on surgical risks.

➢ http://www.breastimplantinfo.org/ what_know/having_problems.html More information on implants.

➢ http://www.breastcancer.org/tre_surg

fearrisks.html This site has good info on surgical risks.

➤ http://www.cancerbackup.org. uk/Aboutcancer/Genetics/Risks-reducingbreastsurgery/Nipple This site explains the options of nipple reconstruction or prosthetics.

➤ http://www.cancer.org This is the home site of the American Cancer Society. Very helpful site and many links.

➤ www.cancer.gov/cancertopics/types/ breast This is the government's cancer web site.

➤ http://www.cancerbackup.org.uk/ Cancertype/Breast/Treatment/Surgery Gives options and information.

➤ http://www.dcis.info/treatment-options. html Explains some of the options of treatment for breast cancer.

➤ http://www.ebreastaug.com/breast-implant/problems.html This site talks about the problems of breast implants.

➤ http://imaginis.com/breasthealth/

<u>pathology2.asp</u> More on pathology reports.

➤ <u>http://www.info.cancer.ca/e/glossary/M/ Multifocal/htm</u> This site has good explanations.

➤ <u>www.komen.org</u> Site specifically for breast cancer. Good reference.

➤ <u>www.nlm.nih.gov/medlineplus/ breastcancer.html</u> Additional governmental site.

➤ <u>http://www.medterms.com/script/main/ art.asp?articlekey=31789</u> Good site for understanding the terminology and also for spelling.

➤ <u>http://www.oncolink.org/books/chapter. cfm?b=21&c=7</u> More information about DCIS.

➤ <u>www.nationalbreastcancer.org</u> Self explanatory.

➤ <u>http://www.thebreastcancersite.com</u> Self explanatory.

➤ <u>http://www.thebreastcancersite.com/</u>

cgi-bin/WebObjects/CTDSites   More information on breast cancer.

➢ http://www.thebreastcaresite.com/EEndCom/USAmoena/Homepage.nsf/1989cec9be30ee68c12569ff0036969d/ff5633aad90dee6a05256ac20059dde8?OpenDocument This is further information on pathology reports.

➢ http://www.xeloda.com/learn-about-diagnosis/breast-cancer/breast-cancer-pathology-reports.aspx This site has a great example of margins.

➢ http://www.y-.org/publications/generalpubs/read_pathology_report.pdf This site is a guide to your pathology report. It has a simple yet very useful 8 page guide on how to read and understand a pathology report.

www.ingramcontent.com/pod-product-compliance
Lightning Source LLC
Chambersburg PA
CBHW052244290526
45785CB00016B/1290

9 7 8 1 4 4 9 7 9 2 0 8 4